Prevention and Care of
ALZHEIMER'S DISEASE

A Practical Guide to Reducing Your Risk, Slowing the Progression and Living with Dementia

LAVONNE STECKBECK R.N.

Prevention and Care of Alzheimer's Disease:
A Practical Guide to Reducing Your Risk, Slowing
the Progression, and Living with Dementia

ISBN-10: 1-4611-7025-7
ISBN-13: 978-1-4611-7025-9
LCCN: 2011907706

PWS Publishing
101 S. E. 6th Court
Pompano Beach, FL 33060 U.S.A.
Email: lsteckbeck@gmail.com
Website & Blog: www.alzheimerspracticalguide.com
Become a Fan on Facebook: www.facebook.com

DEDICATION

This book is dedicated to the loving memory of my husband, Perry Steckbeck. Perry, without whom this book would not have been written, was a man who believed in finding the cures for many diseases. He would appreciate me helping other families meet the challenges we endured together, as well as helping families reduce the chances of ever being diagnosed with Alzheimer's disease.

CONTENTS

Foreword i

Acknowledgments iii

Introduction v

**PART I: A Look into My
Experience with Alzheimer's.........................1**

Perry's Story... 3

Total Control and Brainwashing 15

Neglect.. 21

Stranger in Need... 25

A Different Approach 27

**PART II: What I Have
Learned Since Perry's Passing 33**

Research 35

What Is Being Done Now 39

Prevention with Diet and Exercise.................. 51

Caregiving.. 67

Care for the Caregiver 85

Elder Abuse and Financial Exploitation......... 89

**PART III: When Home Care
Is No Longer Possible 99**

How to Choose a Facility 101

Hospice.. 107

My Plan For the Future................................ 111

Conclusion 115

FOREWORD

Alzheimer's disease (AD) is now recognized as the most common cause of late-life type of dementia throughout the world. Considering the baby-boomer factor, easily we can predict AD to become an overwhelming public health issue by the year 2050. The national financial burden would jump from sixty billion dollars to one hundred billion dollars annually. As a nation, we need to prepare ourselves to confront this disease.

Mrs. Lavonne Steckbeck, a retired nurse and wife who Acquired first hand knowledge of AD while caring for her husband, takes the reader through a journey of where we were, where we are, and where we are heading with this disease. This work is not only an eye-opener but also a guide for anyone who has been touched directly or indirectly by AD. Lavonne writes with such a personal touch that you can't help but to get drawn in into her stories.

Lavonne's professional background as a registered nurse and educator comes through in this excellent work. This is must-read material for anyone dealing with AD, including those at an academic level.

Andy Mencia, MD, CMD

ACKNOWLEDGEMENTS

I want to thank all of my children, Linda, Sandy, Pam, Pete, Bill, Julie, Paul, Mary, and Jeff. Thank you for giving me support in writing this book so other people can meet the problems of taking care of their family members who are faced with this condition. You were with me all the way in taking care of your father with a love like no other. I could not have endured those many years without your help. May this book be a way of helping other families find an easier way to cope with all of the challenges we faced. I love you all so very much.

I would also like to acknowledge Dr. Andy Mencia, MD, CMD, of the Adult and Geriatric Institute of Florida, Inc. Many thanks go out to him for his encouragement to write this book and find answers to the many difficulties we are facing today, in caring for Alzheimer's individuals at home and in extended care facilities. I truly appreciate his input.

I want to give special thanks to Paul Steckbeck, my son, who initially motivated me to write this book. He and his daughter, Allie, helped me organize my thoughts when I needed a direction.

I also want to give special thanks to Jeff Steckbeck, my son and mentor in completing this manuscript to its finish. I certainly needed all his knowledge in choosing the right words. I am thankful for his guidance in writing this book.

My daughter, Mary Steckbeck, RPh, deserves special thanks as well for helping me with the complexities of drug names and reactions. Mary has kept me objective in my portrayal of how drug companies are working diligently for a cure for Alzheimer's.

Joseph Yanero deserves special thanks as well for his genius ability with the computer and my home network. He never gave up on me when I had to ask ridiculous questions about my computer, which my granddaughter knows more about than I do.

INTRODUCTION

I first had the idea to write this book while I was living in a condo I moved into shortly after my husband, Perry, died. I became aware of the lack of attention paid to an obviously confused and possible Alzheimer's person by her own family. Many times patients with Alzheimer's disease are not treated fairly. I was shocked by two such cases that were reported in a South Florida newspaper. It is bad enough that these people have to go through a confusing lifestyle every day, but to be taken advantage of emotionally and financially to me is appalling. So much is known today about Alzheimer's disease that there is no reason a family member cannot get help or knowledge about how to care for a family member with dementia or Alzheimer's.

This brings us to defining the condition. What is Alzheimer's disease, really? I recently had a person ask me this very question. According to my extensive research, it is a group of symptoms marked by certain brain changes. Alzheimer's is not a normal part of aging. It is not something that inevitably happens in later life. The cause is a mystery, which is what is challenging the medical community as well as drug research communities trying to develop a cure. Although Alzheimer's is not curable or reversible, there are ways to reduce the risk, slow the progression, and alleviate the suffering of the individual with Alzheimer's as well as the family.

An analysis of Alzheimer's patterns around the world found that 13 percent of Americans sixty-five and older have Alzheimer's disease. This number is expected to rise dramatically as 2010 saw the first year of the baby boomer generation turn sixty-five. Every seventy seconds, someone in America develops Alzheimer's. By 2050, someone will develop the disease every thirty-three seconds.[1]

Today, doctors are more likely to know when a person has Alzheimer's because of what has been discovered from their symptoms, but still they can only say that it is possible or probable. During the time I was taking care of Perry, the only thing the doctors would tell me was to "get his legal papers in order." Do you know how devastating that was to hear? Well, being one to never give up, I was determined, since I was a nurse, to find a physician who could give me a better prognosis. But after many visits to our primary care physician, a neurologist, psychologist, and even a psychiatrist, who by the way seemed to know very little at the time about Alzheimer's disease, the prognosis was no different.

There are three main parts to this book. The first part is about historically how Alzheimer's individuals were incorrectly diagnosed, cared for, and treated by doctors, families, and the community due to the lack of knowledge about Alzheimer's—and sadly, how Alzheimer's disease individuals were taken advantage of because of this fact.

The second part of this book is what I have learned since Perry's passing in 1997, and the research being done now for this disease. I will also cover some education of my readers as to how to reduce the risk of getting AD in the first place, as well as how to slow the progression of it after the original onset.

The third part is about what happens when home care is no longer possible and the family needs to search for a facility that can take over the care. I will outline my plan for the future caring of Alzheimer's individuals.

I am not a doctor nor am I an authority on what the scientific community is presenting today about the brain and the latest discoveries and about how the AD brain is affected. I am only interested in how we as a society can provide the best care we can to make life with Alzheimer's disease easier, both for the individual with the disease and for the family members.

PART I

A Look into My Past with Alzheimer's

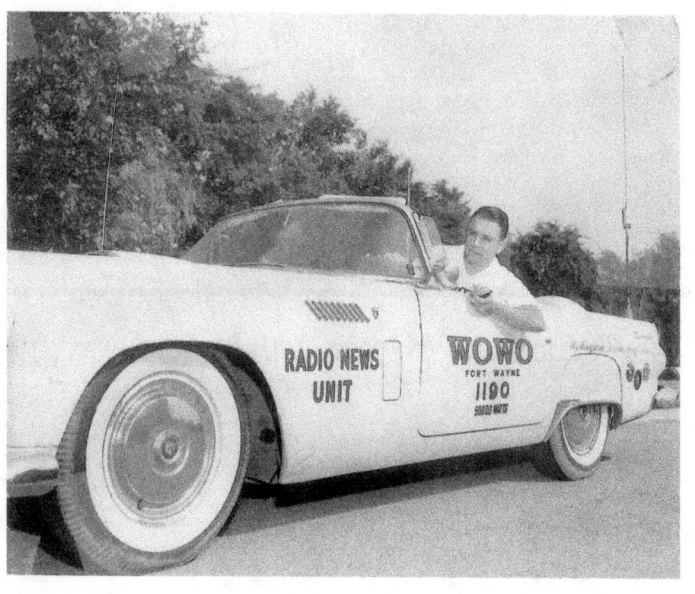

PERRY'S STORY

My husband, Perry, was a very dynamic person who had a personality that just seemed to attract people. . This began when he was in high school. He was voted "friendliest person" in his senior class. The saying was "Perry never knew a stranger." Whomever he met became a friend for life. After getting out of school and after being honorably discharged from the US Army, he worked in the retail paint and wallpaper business with his father in Fort Wayne, Indiana, where both of us grew up and lived.

One day one of his many friends asked Perry if he would like to work for a local radio station, WOWO, also located in Fort Wayne. This job required him to work on-air from eight p.m. to ten p.m. weekly. He would travel around town during the evening in a flashy new Thunderbird Mobil

3

Unit interviewing people for the evening radio show, called Program PM, on anything newsworthy that was going on around town. He even interviewed a man shortly after he delivered his own baby at home.

People got to know Perry traveling around town and called him to get their story on the air. This seemed to fit Perry perfectly because talking to people was what he loved.

After a while, and changing times, another friend asked him if he would like to be a salesman for Motorola Communications, selling two-way radios. This was a dream job for Perry because he loved communicating this way and was a "born salesman" as some called him.

As most people know, the pressure is "on" constantly for anyone in sales, even for someone who found it easy to get business. Eventually this job did take a toll on Perry and he had a brain-stem stroke. This happened when he was forty-nine years old. Even though he had no obvious paralysis or brain damage, he was not the same ever again. He became very depressed because while he was off work, recuperating, he constantly thought his boss was out to take all of his business away from him (a condition called delusion). In fact, his boss was only handling his customers until Perry got back to work.

At this time I do want to interject one fact that could or could not be a contributing factor in Alzheimer's disease, which is head trauma. The Alzheimer's Association currently states that severe head injuries have been associated with increased risk for later development of Alzheimer's disease and other dementias. [5]

When Perry was a teenager, he was hit in the head with a baseball bat during neighborhood play. As the story goes, his mother called the doctor and was told to put ice on the knot and if he was thinking clearly, then he was OK. The doctor did not even suggest having an X-ray done. Thank goodness today more is known about head injuries, and doctors are recommending better and more immediate attention.

After Perry recovered from his brain-stem stroke and went back to work, he did not seem to handle the pressure as he once did. One day he asked me, "What is the name of that street over there, you know, the one that's a bridge?" Well, this was a street he traveled many times a week called Southern Boulevard, in West Palm Beach, Florida, near where we lived at the time. At this point, I began to notice more distinct symptoms of memory lapses and lack of clarity in his thinking. For a person who really did not like going to the doctor, because he thought he was so healthy, I did manage to convince him to go to our primary care physician for a checkup. This was the beginning of our journey with doctors. The first thing we found was that Perry had mild diabetes. He was put on medication for it, and was instructed to take it every day.

Also, at that time Perry was given a short memory test by his primary care doctor. He was given a set of very short obvious questions in series, like, what day is it, and who is the president? He unfortunately failed this test and was given a referral to a neurologist. After that, he was referred to a psychologist and even a psychiatrist. Like I stated before, even the medical community did not know much about Alzheimer's disease in the mid 1980s. Since I was a nurse, I was determined to find the right doctor to treat Perry so he would recover. Some people call this false hope or denial. But I did not think it could be Alzheimer's disease, since he was only fifty-five years old.

As time went on, Perry became more agitated. He could not get out words out he was trying to say, yet he could hear and somewhat understand what we were saying. It was like what he was trying to say was on the tip of his tongue. We were cautious of not speaking about him in front of him, because we knew he still predominately understood what we were saying. This symptom is called "expressive aphasia." Perry became angry with the speech therapist who was trying to help him. My husband was a man who built his whole life around the beautiful meaning of words and talking to people. It was so painful for him that he did not continue speech therapy. Learning how to form the words was not the answer. (There is now an association called the National Aphasia Association, which was founded in 1987, three years later. I have provided information in the resources section of this book.)

One doctor prescribed sertraline and later lorazepam, which neither one helped much and might have made the situation worse. Perry also was given phenytoin, although I don't know why, as it is an antiseizure medication, and he never had any seizures.

Since Perry was not able to work and we had a family to take care of, I went to work and hired a sitter for him. I worked nights because he seemed to sleep well at night. When he eventually needed more care, I placed him in what I thought was the best nursing home in town. Later on, that proved to be untrue. One day, when he became so agitated and of course could not talk to say what was bothering him, he was taken to the Emergency Room of the nearest hospital. I arrived when he was being put in the elevator. Since being in closed spaces seemed to make matters worse, it took four people to hold him down. This was followed by him almost tearing up a room in the ER, and it took six people to hold him down. He was given an immediate injection of haloperidol, a powerful antipsychotic drug. Once he calmed down, he was sent back to the nursing home. Well at that point, I quit work and took him home to take care of him myself. He was given a prescription of this medication when he went home. This started a cycle of hollering and hallucinations that was frightening to watch.

I did not realize it at the time, of course, thinking his hallucinations and delusions were just part of his condition, but I believe now that this drug was possibly the cause of his constant hollering and hallucinations. For example, he would yell, "Fire, fire...call the fire department!" with a look in his eyes as if the fire was actually coming right at him. That was about all he ever said, as he was still suffering from aphasia that seemed to get worse every day. One day, when I went to get this prescription of haloperidol refilled, the pharmacy was out of it and was not going to get it for another twenty-four hours. Well, let me tell you that the next twenty-four hours were the quietest twenty-four hours I had in a long time. Needless to say, I did not pick up that prescription.

I have found out since then that the makers of the drug are no longer recommending it for dementia individuals. How many people like Perry and I had to go through this trauma before they finally decided this was not working and in fact it might have made his condition worse? I am sure we were not alone on this journey, though it surely seemed like we were.

Moving to the end of this story, Perry developed medical problems and needed surgery, which was another traumatic situation. After he came home from this surgical stay, he refused to eat, move, or anything else. He finally passed away peacefully shortly thereafter. I believe he was just tired of the daily struggles. He was sixty-eight years old when he died. A diagnosis from a brain autopsy after Perry's death stated "Alzheimer's disease." This did not state as the cause of death, just a diagnosis, which only confirmed what a neurologist told me thirteen years earlier, which was "dementia, probably of the Alzheimer's type."

Now maybe you can see why I never wanted to have anything to do with Alzheimer's disease again. It took me almost five years to realize this. It took me almost five years to realize how wrong I was. The public needs to know all about Alzheimer's, even the tough part, so we can conquer it and not let it get the best of us.

I am going to stick my professional neck out here and state what I believe was also happening. I believe Perry was also suffering from another dementia condition known as Lewy body dementia. I had never heard of this until about three years ago. No doctor has ever suggested this to me.

According to the Lewy Body Dementia Association Web site, one can have this disease along with Alzheimer's. One of the symptoms of Lewy body dementia is frequent hallucinations and a hypersensitivity to antipsychotic drugs, such as haloperidol, which is the drug Perry was prescribed that might have made the symptoms worse. Below is an interesting direct quote from their Web site in the spring of 2011, at the publishing of this book:

While traditional antipsychotic medications (e.g. haloperidol) are commonly prescribed for individuals with Alzheimer's with disruptive behavior, these medications can affect the brain of an individual with LBD differently, sometimes causing severe side effects. For this reason, traditional antipsychotic medications like haloperidol should be avoided.

In regards to his surgery and the immediate decline post-surgery, the following notation makes sense in Perry's case as well:

Be sure to meet with your anesthesiologist in advance of any surgery to discuss medication sensitivities and risks unique to LBD. People with LBD often respond to certain anesthetics and surgery with acute states of confusion or delirium and may have a sudden significant drop in functional abilities, which may or may not be permanent.

In all my experience of taking care of Alzheimer's disease individuals since Perry's death, in hospitals and nursing homes, I have never seen such extreme hallucinations as Perry had. This is why I believe he also suffered from Lewy body disease.[6]

TOTAL CONTROL
AND BRAINWASHING

I experienced the first incident of unfair treatment of a confused individual when I was looking for a place to rent after moving to Florida from Indiana, after my husband passed away. Some of my children lived in South Florida then and still do. This brings me to the story of my landlord at the time.

She was also a Realtor, and one clue to her confusion was when she could not find the key to open the door. What Realtor does not bring the proper key to open the door for a prospective renter? Most people might have given up, but I really wanted to see this place, which was directly on the ocean, so I waited until she found the correct key. Well, needless to say, I liked it and moved in soon thereafter.

I will call my landlord "Sally" for now. Sally seemed to need a friend, and called and visited often, since she lived in the same building. At first, wanting to stay on a business relationship level, I mailed my rent check to her. After a couple of months of not being able to reconcile my checkbook because the checks were not clearing, I asked her if in fact she had received my payments and if she had, why she had not deposited them. She answered, "Oh, didn't I?" She then said, "I will do that tomorrow." Well tomorrow did not seem to come; the situation did not change. The next thought I had was to staple the check to a pink 8 X 10 piece of paper and hand it to her. This still did not work.

Another day, I went to Sally's apartment, located two floors above mine, and knocked on her door. She answered and we spoke a bit. I asked her if I could take her to the bank, thinking that she might have a problem driving her car. While we were talking, she told me she had received a couple of tickets but laughed about it. I thought to myself, *Hopefully she paid them.* She said, "No,

I do not need you to take me to the bank." She then asked me to come in for a while to visit.

Well, it's a good thing that I am an honest person, because all of her banking and personal papers were scattered about in her kitchen and dining table. My pink piece of paper with the check still attached was lying in plain site. She told me that some day she would take care of everything, when she got time. She also said she knew where everything was. I then inquired of her, "Sally, have you had a hard time remembering things lately?" She said, "No, do you think I do?" Well, I skirted around that question by asking her if she had a doctor and had she been to see him lately. She said, "Yes, I have a doctor; he is a dentist."

Believe me, I hope you are never in this delicate situation that I found myself in right then. Knowing Sally had a sister up north, and who visited her occasionally, I was hesitant to interfere with her personal life, other than to offer my assistance if she needed me.

What I learned from that incident is that even at the sacrifice of causing some perceived embarrassment, I should have interfered and offered to take Sally to the doctor or call her sister. I say this, because the situation got worse. As time went on and I moved out because of circumstances, Sally kept calling me and asking me to move back in, which was impossible.

One morning a friend of Sally's who lived out of state called me to tell me that Sally had fallen in the garage the night before. She managed to get on the elevator and up to her apartment, but her leg hurt. The friend then told me Sally had called the security guard, but he could not leave his post to go help her until seven a.m. the next morning. (This was ten p.m. the night before)

This is why condo owners pay high prices for security today? Well, at seven a.m. an ambulance was called and transported Sally to the hospital, where she was found to have a fractured hip. The hospital staff was challenged due to Sally being in such a confused state, having coped with this for the previous nine hours and having no sleep. They had a hard time getting Sally to understand that they had to get consent from her next of kin to do surgery on her. Well, her sister was finally contacted and surgery was performed on her fractured hip.

After this incident, I was there every day helping care for her and assisting her in physical therapy, simply as a friend. She had a hard time understanding the required physical therapy to get her walking again.

Sally's sister was too busy with her business to come to South Florida to see her or even, for that matter, send a card or flower. Possibly she was in denial that Sally had a problem. This exemplifies how families are at a loss when it comes to caring for Alzheimer's individuals.

The next thing her sister did was unbelievable. This is what I am calling "brainwashing" of the Alzheimer's individual. It is so easy to do. Whether or not malice is involved, the individual has no idea what is happening to them mentally, from an external point of view. Her sister started calling Sally on the phone excessively, sometimes every five minutes, and telling Sally to tell me to leave, because "she did not need me anymore." I could not believe this! I thought the sister felt I was getting too close to Sally and might want to get her some medical care for her dementia. This negotiation phase of her sister's mental process was obvious, and there was nothing I could do to change this "brainwashing" her sister was performing on Sally.

Well, Sally did just what her sister instructed her to do and told me to leave. So, I left and did not see Sally again. I found out from another mutual friend that her sister had taken her home to another state, before she had time to even finish her physical therapy or have her stitches removed.

A financial situation might have been a contributing factor. I'm not sure. The situation with Sally is the ugliest form of brainwashing" I have ever seen up close. I wonder how many other cases of "brainwashing" on Alzheimer's individuals are happening today. Probably more than we want to think about.

NEGLECT

One of the reasons that a lot of people are afraid of Alzheimer's is because of the horror stories that come out about how people react to a family member who is diagnosed with "dementia, probably of the Alzheimer's type." I will give you such a story. This might be the worst you have ever heard; at least it was for me. The next story comes from a 2005 article in a local South Florida newspaper.[2]

The article was about a couple who lived in an affluent neighborhood. They brought the wife's mother here to live with them from Austria. Well, it might have turned out better if they had left her in Austria. Someone there might have taken better care of her than her own daughter.

It was reported after her death that the eighty-nine-year-old lady died in a locked room, ventilated only with wood lattice covering a sliding glass door leading to the outside. Pizza box tops were nailed over the room's air-conditioning vents to keep the stench of excrement from spreading through the rest of the home area. The locked room had no electricity. The article went on to say that the maid refused to go in there to clean. Yes, they had a maid. The woman's mother was fed a diet of honey buns and Ramen noodles. The last time I checked, these two items are not high on the nutrition triangle.

At her death, autopsy photos showed a figure withered to eighty pounds and barely recognizable as a human being. It also was reported that these people did not want to spend their inheritance on medical care for her.

In their defense, their lawyers said, "These people suffered 'caregiver fatigue' and they did the best under trying circumstances." Well, in my opinion, if this is the "best" educated, civilized people can do in taking care of a family member, this country is in worse shape than I thought.

There is so much information available to anyone who cares to find out about how to care for aging, demented individuals that I almost did not write this book. I thought surely everyone knew how to go to the library or bookstore to get information, or better yet how to "Google" caring for Alzheimer's individuals. After all, are we not a society that is Googling, twittering, and texting our fingers off about every little detail in our lives to each other? There is one thing that is not written, however, and that is how to feel love for one's own parents, spouses, or any family member who has AD.

To close on this story about neglect, the Austrian's daughter and husband served a five-year sentence in a Florida prison, giving them time to think about what they did to her mother. I believe they were served, even in our prisons, a better diet than Ramen noodles and honey buns.

STRANGER IN NEED

I do not know if I have a sticker on my forehead reading "ask me" or what but sometimes people come up to me in the strangest of places and ask me "odd" questions. One day when I was in the supermarket in the flower department, a lady came up to me and said, "What color do you think would be for a man?" Well, actually, I had never given a man flowers, but I answered, "Blue, I guess." She followed with, "I think I should get some for my mother, too." She added, "She has Alzheimer's and my uncle is taking care of her in her big beautiful house, but he is not taking very good care of her and it is her house!" The conversation continued and I suggested, "If you think she is being mistreated, maybe you should call the police. She replied, "The police have already been there a couple of times, but he tells them she is OK." Well, obviously someone else thought she was not being taken care of so well.

I gave her my phone number and suggested she call me or the Alzheimer's Family Center locally if she needed more help. She never called. I think of her often and wonder how many other people are in the same situation. No one needs to be alone in this journey of taking care of a relative or friend that has Alzheimer's disease. There are support groups that are extremely important for the caregiver of the individual. These are free groups where anyone can get information about what other people are doing in the same situations. In the back of this book, I have included Web sites of various resources in which to gain information and support. I urge everyone with any doubt about needing help to please ask immediately. It can give you a great peace of mind.

A DIFFERENT APPROACH

This is a story not about abuse, neglect, or lack of caring, but just the opposite. I feel it needs to be told, as an example of what to do in these situations, now that we know what not to do. Also, I feel it needs to be told because it offsets all the bad news in newspapers since sometimes they report the good also. This appeared in a South Florida newspaper.[3]

There was a man named Jeff who was a coach and a defensive coordinator for a Florida high school football team. Jeff's wife, Bobbi, had to give up her job as an interior decorator and take on cleaning jobs, which provided more immediate cash, in order to care for her husband, who had dementia. She decided to do this after interviewing dozens of nursing homes. This came as no surprise to me, and it may not to you either.

Jeff was picked up on weekdays by a bus and taken to an adult day care so Bobbi could do a few cleaning jobs. Jeff and Bobbi were both probably a little more fortunate than most, because of his job he had at school. Many friends come to visit with Jeff. They brought him things and had cookouts and watched football with him. Jeff could not always follow the games like he used to, but having people around him kept him calm.

Bobbi knew she had to keep all the doors locked because Jeff had a habit of wandering. But Bobbi did not mind because she knew this was a way of keeping her husband safe.

Wandering is one of the biggest risks for individuals with Alzheimer's disease. In fact, 60 percent of those with dementia will wander at one time or another, according to the Alzheimer's Association.[4] Wandering can occur quickly and it can happen even with the utmost vigilance. Some who care for those with dementia feel that since their loved one has never wandered, there is no need to worry. However, because of the progressive nature of dementia, wandering can begin at any time, and once someone wanders for the first time, they are more likely to do it again. It is never sufficient to tell the person not to go out alone because they will probably not remember. As the disease gets worse, so does the ability to make good judgments.

Consider these ways to prevent unsupervised wandering:

Install new locks on doors and windows. (Early in the disease the person with Alzheimer's may still remember how to unlock the current locks)

Install locks that are out of the line of vision (at the top or bottom of the door).

Place a mirror near the doorway; the reflection of their own face will often stop them from exiting through the door.

Develop indoor and outdoor areas that can be safely explored, allowing them to satisfy their need to wander.

Place night lights throughout the house. Keep them active; encourage movement and exercise to reduce anxiety, agitation, and restlessness; and involve the person in daily activities, like folding laundry or helping prepare dinner. The Safe Return Program, administered by the Alzheimer's Association and law enforcement agencies, is available today in most communities. This is usually in alliance with medic alert programs. (See the resources section for the Web site and instructions on this program.) In addition to the Safe Return Program, in Margate, Florida, a program called Project Lifesaver (www.sheriff.org) is available. A wristband helps locate people with brain disorders who are prone to wandering. This could apply to Alzheimer's patients or even people with autism. The program involves placing a transmitter bracelet, which looks like a watch, on the wrist, which then transmits a signal to law enforcement. When a person is missing, a trained law enforcement person uses a special tracker system to conduct a search. They respond twenty-four hours a day, seven days a week. In this Project Lifesaver program, there is a small monthly fee based on a scale of income. The battery needs to be checked daily and changed monthly by a caregiver. You can check with you local law enforcement agency to inquire if they have such a program in place.

The ultimate provider of this technology is LoJack. It is a project by them named Project Lifesaver International. It is nice to see a program that was effective in saving lives during abductions and car thefts being applied to saving the lives of Alzheimer's patients. So, if your local law enforcement agency is not rebranding this technology with local charitable dollars like Margate, Florida, and its surrounding communities, you can contact the nationwide program directly by visiting their Web site at www.LoJackSafetyNet.com or 1-877-4-FIND-THEM.

There are times when a caregiver can allow an AD individual to wander with supervision. At these times:

Make sure they feel safe and comfortable. Make sure the room or area is not too cold or too hot.

Ensure adequate lighting as to reduce the risk of falls or injury.

Make sure that the area is not too noisy and that there is not too much going on around them.

One of the most important things to remember in taking care of Alzheimer's disease individuals is keeping them socially active, as in Jeff's case. It is therapeutic when friends of people with dementia visit them often rather than forgetting about them because they cannot have a logical, meaningful conversation.

PART II:

What I Have Learned Since Perry's Passing

RESEARCH

In doing research on this disease, I have discovered there are over five million people living with this debilitating condition in the United States alone. The numbers are much larger worldwide, of course. Yes, there are people around the world who deal with the same problems we have.

When I was volunteering at the Alzheimer's Family Center, which I do regularly, we had a booth at a local health fair. A lady backed away from the table, put her hands up in a defensive manner, and said, "Oh, I don't want to know anything about that; I eat a healthy diet and I'm not going to get it." You would have thought we were talking about the plague. Alzheimer's is not contagious, and although we now think eating a healthy diet is just one of the ways to prevent Alzheimer's disease, we cannot say for sure.

It certainly doesn't hurt to know everything else that can help. Hopefully I can clarify a few facts in this book, so we will not be fearful of it anymore and can truly help those living with Alzheimer's, as well as their caregivers and family members.

Alzheimer's disease was first discovered in 1906 by a doctor in Germany by the name of Alois Alzheimer.[7] However, not much was done to find a cure until thirty years ago when scientists and pharmaceutical companies decided to try to develop a medication that would do just that. So much money has been donated to find a cure, but so far they have not found the magic pill. There are ninety-one drugs in trial, as of the printing of this book in the spring of 2011.[8]

According to one study, long-term use of antipsychotic medication could result in the early death of Alzheimer's individuals. In 2008, British researchers randomly assigned 165 Alzheimer's individuals to either continue their antipsychotic treatment regime or to receive a placebo. Eighty-three continued treatment, and the remaining eighty-two were instead given a placebo. The results showed a significant increase in risk of death for patients who continued taking antipsychotic medication.

The difference between the two groups became more pronounced over time, with twenty-four-month survival rates for antipsychotic-treated patients falling to 46 percent versus 71 percent on the placebo and at thirty-six months it was 30 percent versus 59 percent. This means that after three years, less than a third of people on antipsychotics were alive compared to nearly two-thirds taking the placebo.[9]

Dr. Andrew Weil, a renowned author and physician who attended Harvard, stated, "Don't rule out antipsychotic medications for someone who is agitated or disturbed as to endanger themselves or others, but only for patients as a last resort." Also, he went on to say, "They should only be used for the shortest possible time and lowest possible dose."[10]

Scientists and pharmaceutical companies have made some amazing discoveries in treating just about every disease, and I commend them for their work. There are even new drugs and treatments for cancer that were not even thought possible just a few years ago. I have also found that Alzheimer's disease seems to be the only medical condition today most people are afraid of. Why is that? Cancer is also a devastating disease, but you don't see people ashamed of it, like Alzheimer's. They accept it and try to care for people who have it the best way they know how.

WHAT IS BEING DONE NOW

Most professionals and medical personnel are more open now to talk about Alzheimer's disease. They are becoming realistic in the idea that they need to educate their individuals and family members about how to care for a loved one if they are diagnosed with dementia. The general public is living longer due to increased knowledge about preventing and curing disease. The time for moving forward is now—at least in trying to prevent and give better care for Alzheimer's sufferers and stop waiting for that magic pill.

The Alzheimer's Association advocates early screening whenever a family member has the first signs of memory loss or confusion, also known as cognitive impairment. Early screening is crucial according to the Alzheimer's Association and current national studies, because this is when the most can be done to slow the progression of symptoms. Some people put it off so long because they think it cannot happen to their family member or "It's just old age."

Early Screening

Alzheimer's is a set of symptoms that accompanies specific medical conditions, like loss of memory, language difficulties, and recognition. Memory loss must be severe enough to interfere with everyday life. Before we jump to the conclusion that any changes in memory are indicative of Alzheimer's disease, we need to know a little bit more about changes that may not be Alzheimer's disease, such as the following:

Vascular dementia (multi-infarct dementia caused by multiple small strokes or occlusions)

Parkinson's disease

Depression

Thyroid dysfunction

Medication reaction

Alcoholism

AIDS

Vitamin B12 dysfunction

Memory changes that come with normal aging differ in that they do not interfere significantly with a person's ability to function, as with Alzheimer's disease. Early screening can also relieve anxiety about changes in behavior. The earlier the treatment and care, the better the chances are of a favorable response to treatment, the longer the delay of progressive symptoms, and the lesser financial cost overall.

There is no single scientific diagnostic test to detect if a person has Alzheimer's disease; however, tools and criteria have been developed in recent years to increase accuracy of clinical diagnosis of Alzheimer's disease to 85 percent to 90 percent. Some of these tools are:

Medical history

Mental state evaluation

Physical examination

Neurological examination

Brain scan (CT scan)

Laboratory tests

Symptoms to Watch for Before Going to Your Primary Care Physician

Short-term memory loss of events or learning during events that have taken place within a few hours previous

Problems with language or "finding the right word"

Changes in mood or behavior; signs of depression or uncharacteristic fears of new or unknown situations

Problems with abstract thinking: how to handle balancing the checkbook or paying bills, trouble following instructions or discussion, etc.

Difficulty completing familiar tasks such as preparing meals; stopping in the middle of a significant project, such as making a repair or painting

Disorientation in time and place; wandering and getting lost in places they know well.

Misplacing items, losing things often, or items turning up in unusual places.

Poor or impaired judgment, questionable discussions about money management, or odd choices regarding self-care

What Is the Difference?

Someone with Alzheimer's symptoms:

Forgets the whole experiences (especially recent events).

Rarely remembers later.

Is gradually unable to follow written or spoken directions.

Is gradually unable to use notes.

Is gradually unable to care for self.

Someone with normal age-related memory changes:

Forgets part of an experience.

Often remembers later.

Is usually able to follow written or spoken directions.

Is usually able to use notes.

Is usually able to care for self.

SENIOR MOMENTS

(By the Alzheimer's Family Center, Margate, FL)

Speak to anyone over fifty and they will share with you stories about memory glitches. It is even more evident in people over sixty-five and in still a much larger portion of people over eighty.

You never misplaced your glasses as much as you do now or forget where you put your keys; or worst of all, you could be in the middle of a sentence and the word you are looking for is not on your tongue, a word you use all the time.

There are so many jokes about "Senior Moments," but it is not a joke at all; it can be very embarrassing. There is always the fear of Alzheimer's setting in. Studies have proven, however, that a memory lapse does not mean dementia.

Many times these lapses are "brain busters" stemming from fatigue, depression, poor physical health, and many times from the medications we take. Most of all, stress is the most important factor in memory loss. When you are under a lot of tension, it activates a brain protein called kinase C, or PKC, that can undermine short-term memory. Also the hormone cortisol can damage a part of the brain that is central to memory.

Human memory stores facts, figures, knowledge, and our past and present life as well. It is an autobiographical memory such as the memory of birth(s) in your family, a first kiss, a cruel sight or painful event, or extreme physical pain, which is tied to the human perception of time.

After the ages of forty or fifty, time lasts but a fraction of the time it used to when we were twenty or thirty years old. The whole day seems to speed by, but the hours and days seem to remain the same. This happens because, as philosopher Jean-Marie Gyau's theory states, that memory stores sharp, intense impressions only.

When we were younger we were absorbed in so many new events and happenings each day and looking back over an entire year; it seems long and significant because it was filled with these firsts frequently.

As we age, we have fewer experiences that are dramatic enough to go into long-term storage. Although the days are pleasant at forty, fifty, or sixty and above, we have been there and done that and repeat our daily events over and over again. One week can be just like the next, and then we ask ourselves, "Where did the year go"?

There are ways to improve your memory and to help you remember what you are starting to forget. According to the above philosopher, if you fill your days with as many new and exciting things such as interesting long and short journeys and events to do as firsts again, you will rejuvenate yourself by breathing new life into the world around you. Try to do something different, small or big, each new day. When you look back, you will notice that the incidents heaped up. All those new memories will make the year feel like a year used to feel. It will be a long stretch of time marked by firsts and new experiences and places, thus creating less and less Senior Moments.

Silver Alert

Fred Perry, an Oklahoma state representative, introduced a bill in 2005 that mirrored the "Amber Alert," for seniors in his state called the "Silver Alert." This bill was passed, and it was the catalyst that started a program that has now been adopted by over twenty-seven states. There is much discussion at the Congressional level about whether states should have various levels of alert for different ages of people in our society and situations, and how states can integrate their missing person alerts.[11]

When the Silver Alert for an eighty-six-year-old Boynton Beach, Florida, man with Alzheimer's disease was activated in 2009, the missing man was found safe and sound. This has proven to work many times over in the state of Florida and is very effective at serving as a community safety net for the citizens of the state of Florida.

For families of a senior with dementia, it is important to recognize the risks and try to be prepared. Authorities strongly recommend that families and facilities caring for someone with dementia keep a file containing a recent photo of the person that can be given to authorities if that person goes missing. The file should also contain phone numbers for local police, relatives, and neighbors.

PREVENTION WITH DIET AND EXERCISE

Diet

While we are waiting for a drug to prevent or cure Alzheimer's disease, we can do many things to keep our brains healthy and possibly prevent or at least delay the onset of the disease. I will stress that eating a particular diet will not totally prevent Alzheimer's disease.

The easiest way I have discovered is to keep your heart healthy. It is so obvious, but most people never even think that the blood circulating in our hearts continues up to our brain. Keeping our hearts healthy automatically keeps our brains healthy. Thank goodness a lot of people are doing just that, trying to prevent heart disease by eating a healthy diet and exercising more so they can live a longer life.

Smoking and drinking are also a risk factor for Alzheimer's disease. A study of 938 people by researchers at the Wren Center for Alzheimer's at Mount Sinai Medical Center located in Miami Beach revealed that smoking and drinking are among the most important preventable risk factors for Alzheimer's disease. Are not these the same risk factors for coronary heart disease? People who smoke a pack or more of cigarettes daily develop Alzheimer's more than two years earlier than those who do not smoke. People who have more than two alcoholic drinks a day develop Alzheimer's disease almost five years sooner than people who drink more moderately.

The one diet that seems to pop up most frequently now is the Mediterranean diet. It is called this because the foods this diet recommends are traditionally grown or produced in an area surrounding the Mediterranean Sea. A study reported by CNN in July 2010, performed by Dr. Nikolaos Scarmeas, a neurologist at Columbia University Medical Center and lead author, stated that eating a diet rich in healthy fats and limiting dairy and meat could do more than keep your heart healthy. It could also keep you thinking more clearly by lowering the risk of having small areas of damaged brain tissue or brain infarcts (occlusions). Scarmeas also pointed out that people who most closely followed a Mediterranean diet were 36 percent less likely to have areas of brain damage, compared to those whose eating habits were furthest from this diet. Well, a 36 percent chance of not having brain damage sure is a lot better than anything we have so far!

The Components of a Mediterranean Diet

A substantial amount of nuts, olives, and especially olive oil

An abundance of locally grown fruits, vegetables, and legumes (Who knew we would finally find a good reason to eat all of our vegetables!)

Whole grains, lots of fish, and very little red meat

Low amounts of sugar and saturated fats

Superfoods for Your Brain

According to Dr. Mark Hyman, MD, of the Ultra Wellness Center in Lenox, Massachusetts, and a leader in the nutrition field, you can prevent Alzheimer's disease, boost memory, and sharpen memory by eating smart. Research shows that some foods can improve mental performance and help prevent long-term brain damage. Here are the best choices:

Sardines are recommended in the amount of three cans per week.

Omega-3 eggs are among the best brain foods because they contain folate along with Omega-3s and choline. Folate is a B vitamin strongly linked to mood and mental performance. Eat up to eight eggs a week, but only buy eggs that say "Omega-3" on the label.

Low-glycemic carbohydrates such as chickpeas, beans, soybeans, lentils, and whole-grain breads slow the release of sugars into the bloodstream and prevent sharp rises in insulin that are associated with dementia and damage to blood vessels as well as neurons. The damage is so pronounced that some researchers call Alzheimer's disease "type 3 diabetes." Always eat natural, minimally processed foods, such as apples instead of applesauce.

Nuts such as walnuts or macadamia nuts are the highest in omega 3s, but all nuts are beneficial. Enjoy one to two handfuls daily and avoid highly salted and roasted nuts.

Cruciferous vegetables like broccoli, Brussels sprouts, cauliflower, and kale contain components that help the liver eliminate toxins. One cup daily is optimal, but four cups weekly should be minimal.

B12 vitamins are found only in meat, dairy products, and seafood and are vital for brain health. Two to three daily servings of organic lean meat, low-fat dairy, or seafood are recommended. Dr. Hyman advises everyone to also take a multi-nutrient supplement that includes all the B vitamins.

Green tea is a powerful antioxidant and anti-inflammatory that additionally stimulates the liver's ability to break down toxins. Drink one to two cups a day.

Berries are wonderful foods, especially blueberries, raspberries, and strawberries. The darker, the better. Enjoy one half cup daily of frozen or fresh.[12]

James Joseph, PhD, director of the Neuroscience Lab at the USDA Human Nutrition Research Center on Aging at Tufts University in Boston, says that spinach and strawberries promote signals between cells in the brain, encouraging them to communicate and enhance memory. As we know, Americans have a higher risk of getting Alzheimer's disease, as high as four times the likelihood than in other areas of the world, particularly parts of India. Indian food is commonly known to frequently have high concentrations of curry spice. Researchers at UCLA believe that curcumin found in curry wards off Alzheimer's by preventing the growth of amyloid plaques, sticky proteins that are toxic to brain cells. Curcumin protects us from harmful free radicals, which attack our cells after we metabolize the oxygen we breathe.[13]

Vitamin D

According to David Lee, PhD, research associate at University of Manchester, New England, Vitamin D can boost brain health as well as bone strength. This vitamin, produced when the body is exposed to sunlight and found in foods such as oily fish, seems to preserve mental agility as people age. Possibly it does this by protecting neurons in the brain. Not all studies have found this effect, but vitamin D supplements are also found to protect against cancer and other diseases, so they may be worthwhile in any case. Ask your doctor for more information.

Diet Awareness for Stroke
Victims with Dementia

I do want to mention here what happens when a person has a stroke or heart attack. The person is usually put on a regime of a blood-thinning agent, called warfarin. This is to keep the arteries clear and prevent another occlusion, stroke, or heart attack.

The Mediterranean diet contains lots of green leafy vegetables like lettuce, spinach, broccoli, just to name a few. Consumed in large amounts, these vegetables counteract the actions of warfarin, so it is best to maintain a consistent intake of these and neither avoid nor overindulge. I became very much aware of this while volunteering for a person who has dementia from a vascular occlusion. His wife was having difficulty keeping up with a balanced diet for him that was both healthy but did not unknowingly interfere with the blood-thinning mediation. So checking with your doctor is very important when considering a diet if you or your loved one has dementia from a vascular occlusion.

Exercise

Like I mentioned earlier, it is a good thing a lot of people are interested in being fit these days. Either they want to be healthier and more active or they just want to look good, but either way, the spike in interest in exercising certainly will statistically reduce the number of Alzheimer's cases.

The benefit of exercise, of course, is a healthier heart, and along with this goes a healthy brain. For those not doing any exercising, walking is one of the easiest ways to start. Simply make sure you have comfortable shoes and socks. Exercise can also improve balance and leg strength, which can prevent one from falls. Whether someone is elderly or not, caution should be used when taking medication that can cause dizziness or disorientation. For those who live alone, it is a good idea to have a friend or family member go along. Be sure to hydrate yourself by drinking plenty of fluids, preferably just water, before, during, and after walking. Thirty minutes a day is a good goal to work up to. A study funded by the National

Institute on Aging showed that exercise, particularly walking, can be highly beneficial to elders with severe mobility problems.

Mild Alzheimer's disease individuals with higher physical fitness regimes had larger brains compared to mild Alzheimer's individuals with lower physical fitness levels. When examining this notion further, people with early Alzheimer's disease who were less physically fit had four times more brain shrinkage when compared to normal older adults than those who were physically fit. Therefore, people with possible early Alzheimer's disease may be able to preserve their brain function for a longer period of time by exercising regularly and potentially reducing the amount of brain volume lost.

Evidence shows decreasing brain volume is tied to poorer cognitive performance, so preserving more brain volume may translate into better cognitive performance. This was one of the first studies to explore the relationship between cardiorespiratory fitness and Alzheimer's disease. Just another reason to exercise for the people that need scientific proof!

People who exercise at least twice a week in middle age are less likely to develop Alzheimer's disease when they got older. Walking and cycling are the most popular exercises. Exercise may decrease the risk of developing Alzheimer's disease by improving blood flow to the brain and the transmission of brain signals.

I took care of a lady who only liked to watch TV all day long. She refused to do anything else, her daughter said. Well, after a few days of me volunteering to spend four hours per day with her, I had had enough of following the "soaps." I said, "Next time I come we are going for a walk." She replied, "OK." Well, to my surprise, the next time I arrived to see her, she was dressed and in her walking shoes and ready to go. It was not hard at all to encourage her to walk. She was actually looking forward to it. So all it takes is a little encouragement from a friend or relative. And she did not even mind missing her soaps once a week when I came.

So, start walking, swimming, or whatever exercise you choose. Taking control of your health begins with getting moving! The only days you do not have to exercise are the days you do not eat.

Here it is worth mentioning a true American hero and example of how people should live their lives when it comes to diet and exercise. Francois Henri LaLanne, aka Jack LaLanne, passed away at ninety-six! He refers to the bloodstream as a "river of life which is polluted by junk foods, loaded with preservatives, salt, sugar and artificial flavorings." He often said, "I can't die, it would ruin my image."[14] He certainly did not get dementia. Unfortunately he died of respiratory failure from pneumonia. Well, his legacy will live on in history as being well ahead of his time. Jack knew everything in this chapter a long time ago, and he lived it. He encouraged the elderly to exercise and he ignored doctors telling him that lifting weights could cause a heart attack. Jack also complimented his life with eating healthfully. He's a great example for us all.

Strategies for Healthy Brains

Protect your head: The connection between the development of Alzheimer's disease and previous head trauma is real. Protect your head whenever possible by wearing a helmet while cycling. Always use a seatbelt in a moving vehicle. Also avoid falls by using caution when standing on ladders.

Protect your heart: Everything you do for your heart's arteries, such as controlling blood pressure, cholesterol, and sugar, is good for your brain's arteries also.

Protect your youth: Healthy aging is important for maintaining a healthy brain. Exercise regularly at an early age. Habits formed early on in life usually last later in life. Stay intellectually and socially engaged to improve your brain health, as well as your general health! Remember, age is merely a number!

Mental Stimulation

Mental workouts can be as important as staying physically active. The brains of people in their sixties and seventies who played video games not only remained more agile but showed improved memory and reasoning ability. One of my sons, who sits on the Board of the Commission on Aging for the City of St. Petersburg, says they have a Wii game and a large LCD display in their Sunshine Center in St. Petersburg, where the seniors come for activities. I think this is fantastic.

A new frontier is emerging. Our search for healthier brains has led to the development of software programs and other technology that can improve brain function. Every time we learn something new, our brain grows new tissue. Some things as common as how to program a DVD player or use a new cell phone help keep the brain in condition.

If we could order another helping of brain mass to replace what we perceive is deteriorating daily, mental and emotional stress would be less of a concern. Proper diet, rest, and other factors help maintain the approximately three pounds the human brain weighs. Take a look at how you are processing the things you need to do. By getting your brain to work a little differently, you may find that the drain you experience from daily tasks is because you are doing them the "same old way." The trick is to look at your routine from a new perspective. A change in perspective may make the experience more enjoyable and once again create more of those "firsts" mentioned earlier.

Stay Mentally Active

Do crossword puzzles. Read a section of the newspaper you normally skip.

Socialize regularly. Social interaction helps ward off depression and stress, both of which can contribute to memory loss.

Get organized. You are more likely to forget things if your home is cluttered. Jot down tasks, appointments, and other events in a special notebook.

Focus. Limit distractions, and do not try to do too many things at once.

Drink more water. Not enough water or too much alcohol can lead to confusion and memory loss.

Perform physical activity daily. I cannot say enough about this trait, which increases blood flow to your whole body including your brain.

CAREGIVING

I read an inspiring story about a village doctor in Southern Egypt who was taking care of his own mother with Alzheimer's disease. He stated that you need to cope with the situation one step at a time, and ultimately, until there is a cure, the most we can do for Alzheimer's suffers is to "care for them." Three little words, but with such profound impact!

So many people start out with such high expectations of taking care of their family member with dementia by themselves, but they get weary with all of the stress that comes along with it. For every person with Alzheimer's, it is estimated that there are one to four caregivers involved with their care.

The National Certification Board for Alzheimer's Care (NCBAC) is the first entity to establish itself as a bona fide Alzheimer's care certifying body, by working with another reputable organizations called Meaningful Measurement. The National Certification Board for Alzheimer's Care was eventually born out of the University of Chicago. They confer two credentials, which are "Certified in Alzheimer's Care" (CAC) and "Certified Alzheimer's Educator" (CAEd). In 2006, they had their first pilot tests and certifications and are now the leader in certification of care for Alzheimer's caregivers. I would like to start a school from the proceeds of this book to train health-care workers and certify them in care of Alzheimer's individuals. There are just not enough resources in our communities to train and educate people on the care of Alzheimer's patients.

I recently received an e-mail from a woman sharing her experience of caring for her two parents, both of whom had Alzheimer's disease. In her e-mail she describes her parents as always being very practical due to living through the Great Depression in the 1930s. This woman's mother washed aluminum foil after she cooked in it, then reused it, as an example of frugality and practicality. Her father was happier getting old shoes fixed than buying new ones. Fixing things was a way of life. Sometimes it drove this woman crazy, she mentioned. Just once she wanted to be wasteful. Waste meant affluence to her. Throwing things away meant you knew there would always be more. But then her mother and father passed away. She was struck with the pain of learning that sometimes there isn't any more. Sometimes what we care about most does get all used up and goes away, never to return. Therefore, while we have it, it is best we love it and care for it, and fix it when it's broken.

There are just some people that make life important, such as our aging parents and grandparents. We keep them because they are worth it, because we are worth it. And so, we keep them close.

Gone are the days when a demented person is kept alone in a room and not included in the family activities. Alzheimer's individuals need to remain socially active to keep their brains functioning well.

Have your family member help in preparing part of the meal if they are able to—rinsing the lettuce or setting the table with your supervision. It will enhance their self-esteem and make them feel more valued around the house. They can rinse the dishes, fold clothes, and perform other tasks around the house. These are just small examples of activities that are good for the caregiver and the individual. Someone who is able to go outside can rake the leaves, help with the gardening, or play with the kids in the family.

In a situation where a grandparent is living in a family situation with young children, the children should be taken aside and given a full explanation of their grandparent's behavior. Kids are smarter than we believe sometimes. They want to be included in all activities. It may be hard for the kids to deal with Grandma repeatedly asking the same question over and over, but if they are told ahead of time, the situation will run more smoothly.

Grandparents love to tell stories, and all the children I have known love to hear stories about "the good old days." This can be a wonderful time for both the children as well as their grandparents. It is actually a major part of our culture. Stories shape our culture, and hearing stories of how our grandparents lived helps shape how we act and react to situations, therefore creating a family culture. Looking at photograph albums can also be an opportunity for grandparents to share with the grandchildren. As for teenagers, I bet they did not know that some senior citizens like to watch and even play some of those new computer games out today. The Wii at the St. Petersburg senior center is a great example of that point. If young family members could just spend a few minutes with their older relative with Alzheimer's disease, they might just be surprised what fun everybody can have doing so. And what a wonderful way to keep Grandma and Grandpa stimulating their brains!

Intergenerational schools are in place in some areas of the country. At these schools, young children are brought in to interact with seniors. Dr. Peter Whitehouse, MD,

PhD, a neurologist in Cleveland, has developed such a facility with his wife. He explains this further in his book, *The Myth of Alzheimer's*, which I highly recommend everyone, read. The adult care centers in South Florida have such a program but on a smaller scale. It would be good if a large business or corporation could start something like this in other towns.

Basic Principles in
Understanding and Caring

The Alzheimer's individual is an adult and as such should be treated with respect and dignity even though the behavior seems childlike.

Arguing, confronting, and convincing are counterproductive in dealing with Alzheimer's disease individuals.

The course of the disease and the rate of decline vary with each individual. Everyone is different.

Do not talk about the person as though he or she is not there. Assume the individual can understand what is being said. Do not laugh at inappropriate behavior or speech.

Most people are not intentionally stubborn, mean, suspicious, or ungrateful, nor can they be cured or taught to remember recent events or moral lessons. It is the disease that causes the troublesome behavior.

Creativity and flexibility are necessary in your approach to the person for whom you are caring. If one approach does not work, be ready to try another.

Each task and activity should be simplified and broken into easy steps as much as possible. Reassure the person following each step.

The person becomes more dependent as the disease progresses, requiring increased supervision.

The person functions best in a calm environment with familiar routines of daily living. Eliminate the need for the person to make difficult choices.

Persons with dementia experience reality differently from unaffected people.

Arguing will not change their reality. The technique called "reality orientation" is not effective with persons with severe memory loss, although reminders of time or place may be helpful in making some individuals comfortable. A more useful approach is proactive reminiscence (remembering and discussing past events). Discussing past events that focus on pleasant experiences such as achievement is particularly helpful. This can promote the person's self esteem. Patience is essential when caring for an Alzheimer's individual.

Ten Absolutes

Absolutely Never:

Argue, instead Agree.

Reason, instead Divert.

Shame, instead Distract.

Lecture, instead Reassure.

Say, "Remember," instead Reminisce.

Say "I told you," instead Repeat/Regroup.

Say, "You can't," instead Do What They Can.

Command or Demand, instead Ask/ Model.

Condescend, instead Encourage/Praise.

Force, instead Reinforce.

Loss of Hearing

Loss of hearing is a common problem with elders. But for those with Alzheimer's disease, the situation is much more complicated because the elder may not be able to properly inform you that he or she is having problems with hearing. So, it is up to the caregiver to spot those problems and help correct the situation for the elder. Good communication depends a great deal on being able to hear well. Often enough those people do not themselves know that something is wrong with their hearing. Some things to do when talking to an Alzheimer's person if you suspect he or she has a hearing problem include the following:

Make sure the person can see you well.

Approach the person from the front and face the person directly.

Sit close enough for the person to see your face and mouth.

Keep your hand away from your mouth when you are speaking.

Get and keep the person's attention; wait to begin what you have to say until the person is totally focused on you.

Keep in mind that attention span will be short.

Try to keep eye contact with the person.

If you suspect indeed that your Alzheimer's person has a hearing problem, inform the doctors immediately, so that an evaluation can take place to help make a diagnosis and set up a plan. The doctor will be able to see if the impaired person's hearing is failing or if the problem could be from another source, such as side effects from drugs or the course of the disease itself.

Loss of Vision

Research shows that eye problems are among the most troublesome for elders and can have a very significant impact on their quality of life. Elders with vision problems are:

Three times more likely to become unable to walk.

Four times more likely to develop difficulties eating, dressing, washing, and using the toilet.

Five times more likely to lose their ability to do simple things like taking medication, using the telephone, or managing money.

Vision problems can also lead to increased isolation, depression, and falling. This can be particularly challenging for those elders with Alzheimer's disease because they often cannot communicate that they have an eye problem. So Alzheimer's caregivers need to be especially alert for eye problems and do all they can to get them corrected. Eye problems include anything from diminished vision to serious conditions such as cataract macular degeneration and glaucoma. Studies show that in some cases vision screening methods used in elders are not effective or carried out in the right way. Early diagnosis combined with proper treatment can often save much of the elder's vision. This is why alertness and special training about potential eye problems is a very important part of caregiving.

Depression

Depression is very common among older persons with Alzheimer's disease. It weakens the immune system and makes the person feel overwhelmed by feelings of sadness, helplessness, and worthlessness. This in turn leads to loss of interest in life (social isolation and difficulty in recovery from illness and surgeries.

Fortunately, this illness can be cured if properly identified. Several medications are currently available for treatment of depressive symptoms. Research has shown that depressed elders also need a great deal of emotional support, encouragement, and affection in order to enjoy a better quality of life and eventually recover. A regular program of activities should be considered and can be an amazing benefit in helping elders get over depression. However, depressed elders may be reluctant to become involved and may refuse. Be gentle and do not force them. Just do not forget to show you care for them, and smile.

The Power of a Smile

A smile has amazing power. A smile recognizes a person's worth and is a sign of respect. A smile is a welcoming gesture that invites response and interaction. Everyone in every area of the health-care field needs to understand the power of a smile, especially elder caregivers. A nice smile can be like a ray of sunshine to a lonely or sick elder. They may greatly look forward to your sunny face each day and consider you to be one of the most important people in their lives.

Research shows that facial expressions do affect mood, and a smile is a facial expression—a great one. Smiling makes the person doing the smiling and the recipient of the smile feel happy and experience a positive change in overall mood. Frowning, on the other hand, encourages grumpiness.

Why not smile? There are many reasons people do not smile. Often people don't smile because:

They are too absorbed in what is going on in their own world.

They do not see other people as individuals with their own needs.

They do not think about it.

They do not take the time.

They are too task-oriented and forget about the people around them.

They do not live in and appreciate the moment. They are always looking ahead to what has to be done.

They get tired of trying because people do not respond to their gesture.

Smiling at others is not always easy. Life seems to throw roadblocks and difficult circumstances at us, which sometimes make it hard to remember to smile. Health-care workers especially have to concentrate on smiling because their actions affect those they care for and can influence the person's day-to-day existence and happiness.

A smile is important in caregiving because it:

Acknowledges other's existence and importance to you.

Lets everyone know that things are OK.

Makes people feel good.

Supports self-confidence.

Supports a feeling of self-worth.

Welcomes the person who receives the smile.

Reflects openness and interest.

Forces a "slow-down" to think of someone else and gets us out of ourselves.

Promotes a sense of belonging.

Erases tension.

Makes it hard to be angry, grumpy, or intolerant.

Encourages a smile back.

Helps lighten any burden.

Helps adjust attitudes of both the giver and the receiver.

Offers kindness.

Has the same meaning in all languages and in all age groups.

James M. Barrie once said that people who bring sunshine into the lives of others cannot keep it from themselves. Smiles have the power to bring sunshine, hope, comfort, and a sense of well-being to everyone. Those who reside in health-care facilities need all caregivers to have the power of a smile.

Laughter

It is worth noting some attributes of laughter and how laughter affects the brain. According to Dr. Lee Berk, a professor of pathology and laboratory medicine at Loma Linda University in California, laughter is hearty medicine. It boosts the immune system and triggers a flood of pleasure-inducing neurotransmitters in the brain. Laughter increases immunity to infections by instantly increasing a flood of disease-fighting cells and proteins in the blood. Brain wave activity changes when we catch the punch line of a joke. 15

Dr. Stanley Tan, also of Loma Linda and an expert in laughter's effects on the nervous system and endocrine systems, says humor provides a safety valve that shuts off the flow of stress hormones—the fight-or-flight compounds that come into play during times of stress, hostility, and rage. Stress hormones also suppress the immune system, raise blood pressure, and increase the number of sticky cells called platelets that can cause fatal obstructions of arteries. So, do what these doctors have found and laugh it up! You don't stop laughing because you grow old; you grow old because you stop laughing![15]

CARE FOR THE CAREGIVER

Caregiving is a stressful and demanding job for which there is usually little opportunity for preparation. To deal with this effectively, the realities of coping with the disease must be accepted. Managing dementia is such a major undertaking that it is beyond the resources of a single, unassisted individual. Each situation is different, and caregivers should not judge their own abilities based on the coping abilities of others.

Support groups have proven to be a valuable resource for caregivers. Through participating in a support group, a family member can receive emotional support and the opportunity to share information, feelings, and experiences in coping with the problems of Alzheimer's disease. Participants in support groups have found that there is no problem "too secret" to discuss, no behavior too bizarre to be understood by other members of the group. Much like other support groups for problems relating to addiction or abuse, support groups are proven to work if the participant truly is committed to receiving help.

The well-being of the caregiver requires priority consideration. Thought must be given to the fate of the Alzheimer's individual if the caregiver becomes too emotionally or physically exhausted or ill. Caregivers need to seek professional help if symptoms of depression interfere with their daily functioning.

Knowledge increases understanding and helps prepare the caregiver to deal with the particular problems that are characteristic of Alzheimer's disease. Understanding the disease enables the caregiver to take control and do what must be done.

Social activities for the caregiver provide renewed energy and help normalize the experience of caregiving. Respite from caregiving helps restore energy and maintains caregiving abilities. Caregivers should take advantage of the many places that offer volunteers for a few hours, like the one with which I am associated. It may sound like a short time, but the caregivers I know really enjoy just a few hours when they can relax and take care of themselves for a change.

I recommend creating a support team. Make a list of people who are willing to help you and be "on call" when you need them. Make a "what can I do" sheet listing things you need and ways others can help. When the support team asks, have them choose from the list. No one expects you to do this alone. It is just too much of a task to do without any help.

The National Women's Health Information Center describes these warning signs that should not be ignored:

Not getting enough sleep or sleeping more than you should.

Significant weight changes.

Losing interest in activities that were once enjoyed.

Becoming easily angered or irritated.

The American Heart Association offers these suggestions for caregivers:

Sneak in a ten-minute walk by yourself when possible.

Designate a quiet, peaceful place at home where you can go to relax, pray, read, or enjoy music.

Do not let your loved one discourage your quiet time. Reward him or her after you have had a chance to relax to encourage and support this activity.

ELDER ABUSE AND FINANCIAL EXPLOITATION

Some loving caregivers who are taking care of spouses or parents who have dementia may think it is impossible for anyone to abuse their family member. However, there are many different kinds of abuse, and it does happen, as I have outlined in several cases earlier in this book. Elder abuse is a general term used to describe harmful acts toward an elderly adult, such as physical abuse, sexual abuse, emotional or psychological abuse, financial exploitation, and neglect including self-neglect. Self-neglect signs are failure to take necessary medicine, leaving a hot stove unattended while in use, poor hygiene, confusion, unexplained weight loss, and dehydration.

Elder abuse is an expanding serious problem affecting hundreds of thousands of elderly people in the United States. Since the abuse is often at the hands of a family member or friend, the issue remains largely hidden by the families, causing gross under-reporting of the crisis. It is estimated that only one out of fourteen incidents comes to the attention of authorities. Criminal prosecution rarely occurs, because by the time law enforcement gets involved, the incident has long passed and the family does not want to bring attention to their disgraceful situation. Overburdened caregivers ride a roller coaster of emotions, feeling overworked, out of control, sad, angry, guilty, and obligated to be constantly available.

National Center on Elder Abuse statistics estimate between one and two million Americans age sixty-five or older have been injured, exploited, or otherwise mistreated by someone on whom they depended for care or protection.[16]

You would think that a person who has cognitive impairment might be unable to describe mistreatment; however, that is not the case. Rather than an inability to describe mistreatment, what might stop an elderly person from reporting abuse is a sense of embarrassment or fear of retaliation. To complicate matters, differences exist among cultural groups regarding what defines abuse.

It is no surprise to discover the mortality rate of an elderly person who has been mistreated is higher than the mortality rate of an elderly person who has not experienced abuse. Nonetheless, numerous success stories exist regarding successful intervention. Social workers and health-care professionals, as well as concerned citizens from a variety of backgrounds, have played a key role in identifying and obtaining treatment for abused elders.

The National Center for Elder Abuse reports that 20 percent of caregivers live in fear they will become violent, and this rate increases to 57 percent among caregivers who have previously experienced violence from those they now care for. Elder abuse is an issue that needs to be addressed as closely as domestic violence. Through public awareness and education, another taboo can be brought out in the open, so offenders will think twice before they lash out and abuse. Ideally, they will know to seek the help of a mental health professional long before they cross the line and begin abusing.[16]

Family doctors and therapists should routinely screen their patients for "caregiver burnout" so stress, frustration and depression can be addressed immediately. Elder care workers in the home or in professional settings should be required to undergo extensive criminal background checks.

Anyone who suspects any type of elder abuse must be encouraged to report it immediately. In the back of this book, there are many Web sites and phone numbers for that purpose.

Financial Exploitation

Financial exploitation is the illegal or improper use of another individual's resources for personal profit or gain. This type of exploitation encompasses a broad range of conduct, from deception to intimidation. For example, a friend of mine became the caregiver for her neighbor when the previous person who was taking care of her was found to have written a check for four hundred dollars as a payment on a cruise for herself. This information is for family members, caregivers, or any senior citizens who live alone and want to be in charge of their own finances, as long as they can.

Stay socially active. Social isolation increases your risk of becoming a victim of financial exploitation. Become familiar with the many programs in your community designed to bring people together and to help elderly people and their families. Establish relationships with the professional who handles your money, like your banker, attorney, and financial consultant.

Don't give away property. Before you enter into an agreement for lifelong care, discuss the arrangement with a trusted friend. Document the agreement and specify the compensation if any is expected. And finally, understand what you are signing. Put all financial documents in a safe place. Do not sign blank checks allowing another person to fill in the amount. This may sound obvious to some, but it happens with high frequency in Alzheimer's cases. Do not sign anything you do not understand. Be aware of scams. As the notion goes, "If it sounds too good to be true, it probably is."

Do not give anyone your ATM or PIN numbers. Cancel your ATM card immediately if it is stolen or misplaced. If you find it, that's great, but the risk of it being in the wrong hands are much greater than simply having to wait a few days for a replacement card. Check your bank statements for unauthorized withdrawals.

Planning for the future is one of the best ways to avoid elder abuse and financial exploitation. Consider a variety of retirement options that will encourage safety as well as independence. It is important for everyone to know their rights and be advocates on their own behalf. Elders with Alzheimer's need to get their financial and other personal affairs in order, before the disease advances to the stage where they cannot make these decisions on their own. Basic legal and financial instruments, such as a will, a living trust, and advance directives, are available to ensure that a person's late-stage or end-of-life health care and financial decisions are carried out to their proper expectations when they were made while they were of a sound mind and body. Many times, caregivers and other family members are involved in or witness the changing of these documents when the individual is no longer in this sound state of mind. Then, it usually gets settled in court, which adds much stress and difficulty to an already hurting family and individual. There are many high-profile cases exemplifying this.

Advance directives for health care are documents that communicate the health-care wishes of a person with Alzheimer's disease. These decisions are then carried out after the person no longer can make decisions. These documents must be prepared while the person is legally able to execute them. A living will records a person's wishes for medical treatment near the end of life. It may:

Specify the extent of life-sustaining treatment and major health care the person wants.

Help a terminal individual die with dignity.

Protect the physician or hospital from liability for carrying out the individual's instructions.

Specify how much discretion the person gives to his or her proxy about end of life decisions.

A Durable Power of Attorney for health-care document appoints a designated person, sometimes called an agent or proxy, to make health-care decisions when the person with Alzheimer's can no longer do so. Depending on the state laws and the person's preferences, the proxy might be authorized to:

Refuse or agree to treatment.

Change health-care providers.

Remove the individual from an institution.

Decide about making organ donations.

Decide about starting or continuing life support, and if so, for how long (if not specified in a living will).

PART III:

When Home Care Is No Longer Possible

HOW TO CHOOSE A FACILITY

It is a wonderful thing and an ideal situation if one family member can be the primary caregiver in the home for an Alzheimer's individual. However, sooner or later, especially in the later stages, it is just too much of a burden for that one person and there is no other family member available to take over the job.

If there is more than one sibling involved taking care of a mother or father, there should be a family meeting. It is hard to know where to start. The first step is to get all the family members together. Of course, this is not always possible if the relatives are scattered about the country. Today, we are fortunate to be able to use tools such as Skype, a widely used video conferencing tool available on the Internet at a relatively low cost. Or your family could utilize a conference call to get everyone together to be a part of the discussion.

As I said in an earlier chapter, it is not good to talk about loved ones as though they are not present. It depends upon their medical condition and the family situation whether they should be present and part of the conversation. Maybe the meeting could be held at a place outside of the home. You would have to have a friend to stand in as a caregiver during this time, if you are the primary caregiver.

There are many different options to consider as far as where placement should be. In doing research on this, I found so many different facilities, it is mind-boggling. For many years, there was only one decision to make, and that was which nursing home to choose. Today, that is not the case, thankfully. Consulting with a physician and following his or her recommendations should be the first priority. I will just give general categories to explore because the bottom line here is finances.

According to the Alzheimer's Association's Facts and Figures report in 2011, the cost of caring for a single person with Alzheimer's disease is estimated to be $56,800 yearly. The bulk of this is typically provided by each family. When nursing home placement is necessary, the annual cost rises to $64,000.

Medicare does not cover anything until the Alzheimer's individual must be admitted to a nursing home or skilled nursing facility as a Medicare patient or has a rehabilitation status dictated by their doctor.

In regard to private insurance companies covering facility care for the Alzheimer individual, I am told they typically do not cover dementia care for individuals in facilities, unless there is a policy for this. Insurance companies have so many different options now for this end-of-life care; it really depends on what insurance the individual has. Some private disability policies cover it and some do not. I recommend checking with the Veterans Administration because their policies tend to change.

In most cases, the cost is the burden of the family, and it either comes from the individual's savings or a family member's.

It can range from $1,900 a month to over $4,000 a month, depending on the facility.

Level 1—Independent Living

This is sometimes called "resort style" living. Residents here have their own private rooms with access to three meals per day as well as all the activities and entertainment. Residents are also allowed to go out on their own without checking in or out. Some can even drive their own cars. Also twenty-four-hour medical assistance is provided if needed.

Level 2—Assisted Living

This is a little bit more restricted than the independent living option in that residents need to check in and out when they leave the facility. They need some assistance typically with daily living. They receive three meals per day and are given medical assistance when needed. They can have their own room or a shared room. Also, residents can participate in a full schedule of activities if they care to.

Level 3—Alzheimer's Unit

This is a totally locked unit in an assisted living facility to keep the residents safe from wandering away. Some have shared rooms but are allowed to move about the area as they care to. They may also have a full schedule of activities and a private dining room where they can be assisted with eating if necessary. The nursing aids usually have some special training in taking care of Alzheimer's individuals.

Level 4—Full Nursing Home Care

Nursing homes are sometimes called "Skilled Nursing Facilities," depending on what kind of care the individual needs at the time. They usually have a separate unit away from regular nursing home residents for Alzheimer's individuals. Do not put your loved one with Alzheimer's disease at one of these facilities, as they need to be taken care of in a special way and do not do well otherwise.

Even though there are many excellent nursing homes, most are understaffed and consequently there is a high overturn of caregivers. The reason for this is that they have not been trained specifically for caring for dementia individuals and they become very stressed and leave.

Overmedication of overactive Alzheimer's individuals, even though antipsychotic medications are not recommended, still occurs. This care of the individual is uneducated, often misguided, and sometimes unintentional. Education about drug medication and how to care for the special needs of the Alzheimer's individual is needed.

A friend told me of a time when her mother was so overmedicated she was unable to communicate with her. It can also swing the other way, and the legal community is overzealous in what they think is mistreatment and carry through on unnecessary procedures or lawsuits.

There is a large need for a more powerful patient advocate association to see that these situations do not happen. I have a Web site in the back of this book to help you in choosing a facility.

HOSPICE

Hospice is not a place but a philosophy of care. It is rooted in the belief that everyone deserves peace, comfort, and dignity at the end of life. It is unfortunate that more people do not know about or use hospice. I call it God's gift to the dying. Most caregivers of Alzheimer's individuals do not want to call hospice because they think their loved one is going to die. In fact, that is the truth. However, hospice does not enable a person to die any sooner than they normally would—and what a comfort they can be to the individual as well as the family if called upon earlier instead of in the last month of life! Also they are on call twenty-four hours a day for medical support, and provide trained support specifically for Alzheimer's individuals.

A common myth is that hospice is only for people with cancer. The fact is, hospice is appropriate for patients with any life-limiting illness. Even though I am a registered nurse, I still needed help in dealing with the dying process of my husband. I particularly needed hospice at ten p.m. one night when Perry had a medical emergency. Alzheimer's individuals can keep their primary care physician, but there is a hospice care medical director available for consultation who will make house calls if necessary. The care that is given is called palliative care, described as relief without curing. The goal is to relieve and prevent suffering and to improve quality of life. The care is typically administered by an RN, LPN, Certified Nursing Assistant, social worker, chaplain, trained volunteers, or bereavement specialists. They also provide medical equipment and medications for pain or symptom management.

Hospice is a benefit of both Medicare and Medicaid as well as the Veterans Administration and private insurance carriers. They are typically nonprofit individual chapters around the country, funded by a number of agencies. A key safety net of hospice is that no one is refused care, regardless of ability to pay.

Individuals admitted to hospice care usually have a limited life expectancy, generally six to twelve months. However, if a person lives longer, care will not cease as long as there is a steady decline in their condition. They will be reevaluated every six months. Again, people tend to wait until the last moments because of hospice's reputation as end-of-life care.

Individuals can be cared for by hospice at home, at a hospital, in an assisted living facility, or at a hospice house. When patients are cared for at home, they also educate families on the basics of caregiving. When families need respite after a tiring day, hospice volunteers are there to lend a hand. I have also known people who were in hospice houses with beautiful, tranquil settings. Family can come and go as they please and even stay overnight with the individual. This is often helpful, since many times relatives come from out of town. The care at hospice houses is outstanding.

Bereavement support is another vital service hospice offers. They prepare families for their loss and help them grieve, heal, and embrace life again.

MY PLAN FOR THE FUTURE

The federal government is in such bad fiscal shape today, it is almost impossible to think that we are going to get any help taking care of Alzheimer's individuals. A few years ago, when AIDS was such a major health crisis, it seemed like everyone in the country was having fundraising activities for AIDS sufferers. With more people living longer and with the retiring of the baby boom generation over the next two decades, Alzheimer's disease is going to be as major a medical situation, if it isn't already, as AIDS was previously.

Private funding, either from individuals or large corporations, needs to be spent to educate caregivers and health-care professionals on better care and treatment right now. We cannot wait for pharmaceutical companies or scientists to come up with a medication to cure Alzheimer's disease, if there will ever be one. People have been waiting for a cure, and it still has not been developed.

I would like to see a major corporation start more intergenerational schools like the one Peter Whitehouse started in Cleveland, where seniors can interact with children in an effort to keep their brains stimulated. It can also be a way of helping educate the young people in our society about how to prevent and care for Alzheimer's disease to drastically reduce this disease from becoming a long-term medical problem in the United States.

I am happy to see a program in South Florida schools where they are changing the menus to more healthy food and away from pizza, fast foods, and highly processed foods. If we can get the young sector of our society to eat more healthy food, they will learn to appreciate the true taste of fresh food and carry it over to their adult life. A side effect is that students will be more alert in school.

The ultimate answer will be in generations to come: how they live their lives, the diets they eat, and the exercise they do all throughout their lives, here in the United States, where we have the highest rate of this disease in the world.

CONCLUSION

I had a difficult time bringing an end to this book. I continually kept thinking, "There is more to be told about Alzheimer's disease." However, I believe I have covered the most important facts about the subject. More words would only be repetitive. I believe all of the facts are similar surrounding Alzheimer's disease, and yet somewhat different no matter the situation. The Alzheimer's Association can supply information you may need about any particular situation or location.

My main purpose is to stimulate everyone who reads my words to actively join me in somehow obtaining funds to educate the general public, as well as health-care workers who take care of Alzheimer's Disease sufferers. Above all, do not be afraid of it any longer.

Another fact to remember, as stated in the introduction, is that Alzheimer's disease affects only 10 to15 percent of persons over sixty-five in America. The remaining 85 to 90 percent fulfill their lives with no significant decline in intellectual functioning.

I did briefly mention volunteering. If there is no agency in your town with a leadership role in this, please take it upon yourself to offer your time to someone you know who needs relief in taking care of a loved one with dementia. If I helped only a few people to show more patience and compassion than they ever thought possible in caring for their family members with Alzheimer's disease, I will be happy I wrote this book.

Just remember except for "the Grace of God," Alzheimer's disease could happen to any one of us. Thank you for purchasing and reading this book.

Lavonne

REFERENCES

1. Hebert, L.E., L.A. Beckett, P.A. Scherr, and D.A. Evans. "Annual incidence of Alzheimer's disease in the United States projected to the years 2000 through 2050." *Alzheimer's Disease and Associated Disorders.* 2001;15:169–173.

2. Diaz, Missy. "West Boca couple go on trial accused of starving aging woman with Alzheimer's. At issue: Alzheimer's and in-home care." *South Florida Sun Sentinel.* August 31, 2009; Page 1, 7A.

3. Doup, Liz. "Alzheimer's: A Love Story. Somewhere there's still a little bit of Jeff." *South Florida Sun Sentinel.* January 27, 2008; Page 8G.

4. Alzheimer's Association. "Wandering." Retrieved February 23, 2011, from www. alz.org.

5. Alzheimer's Association. "Stay Physically Active." Retrieved March 1, 2011, from www.alz.org.

6. Lewy Body Dementia Association. "Treatment Options." Retrieved March 2, 2011, from www.lbda.org.

7. *AARP Bulletin*. "The Alzheimer's Century." June 2007. Page 3.

8. The Alzheimer's Association. "91 Drugs Meant To Slow Or Stop Alzheimer's Are Now in Clinical Trials." *Alzheimer's Care Guide*. Sept. 2010.

9. Ballard, Clive (neuroscientist). "Dementia Drugs 'Double Death Risk.'" *Lancet Neurology Today*. January 9, 2009. Press Release April 2009.

10. Weil, Andrew, MD. "Drugs Raising Risks for Alzheimer's Patients." *Self Healing*. March 2009.

11. Holleyman, Summer L. "OK-Representatives plans 'Silver Alert' System for Finding Missing Seniors." iCapitol.net. December 6, 2005.

12. Alzheimer's Family Center. "Superfood for Your Brain." *The Volunteer Vine.* July, August, September 2009, Page 5.

13. Ansel, Karen, RD. "The Anti-Aging Diet." *Family Circle.* August 2008. Page 98.

14. LaLanne, Jack. *Revitalize Your Life: Improve Your Looks, Your Health & Your Sex Life.* Hastings House. 2003.

15. Ricks, Delthia. "Hahahahahahahaha-hahahaaha." *Sun-Sentinel.* November 4, 1996. Page 3.

16. National Center on Elder Abuse. "Elder Mistreatment: Abuse, Neglect, and Exploitation in an Aging America. National Research Council Panel to Review Risk and Prevalence of Elder Abuse and Neglect." 2003. Washington, DC.

RESOURCES AND LINKS

Alzheimer's Association
www.alz.org

Alzheimer's Association Safe Return Program
www.alz.org/SafeReturn

Alzheimer's Disease Education & Referral
Center
www.alzheimers.org

Alzheimer's Disease International
www.alz.co.uk

The Alzheimer's Research Forum
www.alzforum.org/home.asp

The Alzheimer's Resource Room
www.aoa.dhhs.gov/alz/index.asp

The Alzheimer's Family Center, Inc.
www.alzcenter.org

The Alzheimer's Society
www.alzheimers.org.uk

The Alzheimer's Store
www.alzstore.com

ALZwell Caregiver Support
www.alzwell.com

The American Health Assistance Foundation (AHAF)
www.ahaf.org

ElderCare Online
www.ec-online.net/alzchannel.htm

Family Caregiver Alliance
www.caregiver.org/caregiver/jsp/home.jsp

Leeza's Place
www.leezasplace.org

Mayo Clinic
www.mayoclinic

The Nun Study
www.mc.uky.edu/nunnet

PuzzledMinds
www.puzzlemind.com

The Ribbon Online
www.theribbon.com

National Institute on Aging
www.nia.nih.gov

NIHSenior Health
www.NIHSeniorHealth.gov

The National Aphasia Association
www.aphasia.org

New Lifestyles, The Source for Seniors
www.newlifestyles.com
Guide to Senior Housing and Care

www.ingramcontent.com/pod-product-compliance
Lightning Source LLC
Chambersburg PA
CBHW051536170526
45165CB00002B/754